A COMPLETE ALKALINE DIET RECIPES FOR BEGINNERS

Reset and Re-balance Your Diet Through 25+ Wholesome Alkaline Recipes That Will Make Your Life Healthier and Happier!

BY

Urban Robinett

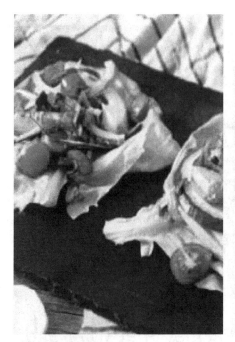
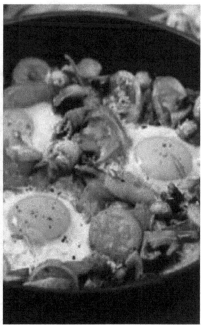
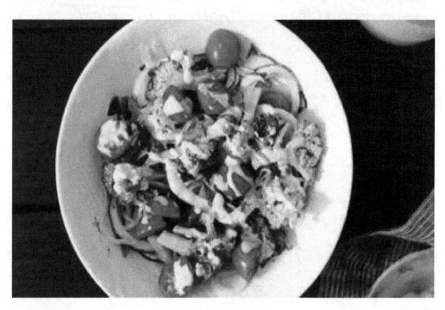

Table of Contents

Conclusion ----------------------------------- **80**

INTRODUCTION

The alkaline diet is very sound, empowering a high admission of natural products, vegetables, and solid plant food sources while limiting prepared lousy nourishments.

Notwithstanding, the idea that the diet helps wellbeing as a result of its alkalizing impacts is suspect. These cases haven't been proven by any dependable human investigations.

A few investigations propose beneficial outcomes in a little subset of the populace. In particular, a low-protein alkalizing diet may profit individuals with persistent kidney sickness

All in all, the alkaline diet is solid since it depends on entire and natural food sources. No solid proof proposes it has anything to do with pH levels.

1. Chorizo hot dogs with chimichurri

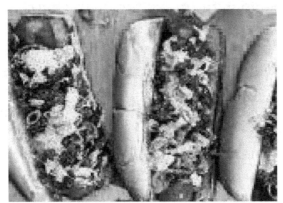

Prep: 15 mins Cook: 25 mins Serves 6

Ingredients:

- 6 chorizo-style wieners or cooking chorizo (not the restored kind)
- 1 tbsp. olive oil
- 6 banana shallots, stripped and cut lengthways
- 3 tbsp. sherry vinegar
- 1 tbsp. nectar
- 6 wiener buns split
- 3 tomatoes, finely chopped
- 50g feta, disintegrated
- For the chimichurri
- 1 banana shallot, stripped and finely chopped
- 1 medium red bean stew, finely chopped, in addition to a couple of cuts to serve
- 1 garlic clove, squashed
- 2 tbsp. sherry vinegar
- Little pack of parsley, finely chopped

- Little pack of coriander, finely chopped, in addition to additional leaves to serve
- 50ml additional virgin olive oil, in addition to 1 tbsp.

Strategy:

1. To begin with, make the chimichurri. Consolidate the ingredients in a bowl with ½ tsp. salt and put away. Will keep for as long as one day in the ice chest. To save money on hacking time, you can likewise barrage the ingredients together in a little food processor until joined however not smooth.
2. Heat the flame broil to medium-high, or light a grill and stand by until the flares have subsided. Put the frankfurters on a foil-lined plate and flame broil for 12-15 mins, or cook on the grill until sizzling and cooked, turning partially through.
3. In the interim, heat the oil in a skillet and fry the shallots for 10-15 mins until delicate and beginning to brown. Mix in the vinegar and nectar and cook for a couple of moments more until tacky.
4. Warm the wiener buns under the flame broil, on a frying pan dish or the grill, and cut the cooked hotdogs down the middle lengthways, in the event that you've utilized short cooking frankfurters. Stuff the buns with the hotdogs, at that point top with a major spoonful of chimichurri, some chopped tomato, the disintegrated feta, some stew cuts, a couple of coriander leaves and the tacky shallots.

2. Stuffed pumpkin

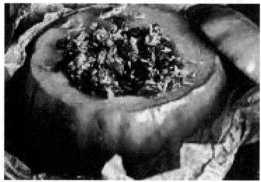

Prep: 15 mins Cook: 1 hr. Serves 4
Ingredients:
- 1 medium-sized pumpkin or round squash (about 1kg)
- 4 tbsp. olive oil
- 100g wild rice
- 1 enormous fennel bulb
- 1 Bramley apple
- 1 lemon, zested and squeezed
- 1 tbsp. fennel seeds
- ½ tsp. bean stew chips
- 2 garlic cloves, squashed
- 30g walnuts, toasted and generally chopped
- 1 enormous pack parsley, generally chopped
- 3 tbsp. tahini
- Pomegranate seeds, to serve

Technique
1. Heat oven to 200C/180C fan/gas 6. Cut the top off the pumpkin or squash and utilize a metal spoon to scoop out the seeds. Dispose of any succinct pieces yet save the seeds for some other time (see our pumpkin seed

formula thoughts). Put the pumpkin on a preparing plate, rub with 2 tbsp. of the oil all around, and season well. Broil in the focal point of the oven for 45 mins or until delicate, with the 'cover' as an afterthought.

2. In the mean time, flush the wild rice well and cook adhering to pack directions, at that point spread out on a heating plate to cool. Daintily cut the fennel bulb and apple, at that point press over ½ the lemon juice to stop them staining.

3. Heat the excess 2 tbsp. oil in a griddle. Fry the fennel seeds and bean stew chips, at that point, when the seeds start to pop, mix in ½ the garlic and the fennel. Cook for 5 mins until relaxed, at that point blend through the apple, walnuts and lemon zing. Eliminate from the heat. Add the combination to the cooked rice, at that point mix in the chopped parsley and taste for preparing.

4. Pack the blend into the cooked pumpkin and get back to the oven for 10-15 mins until everything is steaming hot. Then, whisk the leftover lemon juice with the tahini, the remainder of the garlic and enough water to make a dressing. Serve the pumpkin in the table, finished off with pomegranate seeds and the dressing.

Formula TIPS

Broil THE SEEDS TO MAKE A SNACK

Broil the pumpkin seeds in tamari, maple syrup and stew drops for an exquisite tidbit. Or on the other hand look at more approaches to utilize pumpkin seeds.

Works out in a good way for

Cook potatoes with paprika

Bean stew scorched Brussels sprouts

Thyme simmered vegetables

3. Alkaline Spicy vegetable stew with coconut

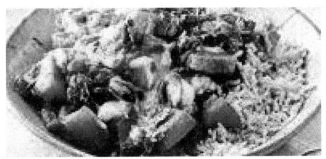

Prep: 10 mins Cook: 40 mins Serves 4
Ingredients:

- 1 tbsp. rapeseed oil
- 2 enormous onions meagerly cut
- 1 tbsp. finely chopped ginger
- 3 garlic cloves, chopped
- 1 enormous red bean stew, deseeded and meagerly cut
- 1 tbsp. thyme leaves
- 1 tsp. cinnamon
- 1 tsp. smoked paprika
- 2 tsp. ground coriander
- 2 tsp. cumin seeds
- 2 x 400g jars chopped tomatoes
- 800ml vegetable bouillon made with 4 tsp. vegetable bouillon powder
- 2 green peppers, cultivated and cubed
- 1 yam, cultivated and cubed
- 2 plantains, stripped and cut
- 160g brown basmati rice
- 2 x 400g jars red kidney beans, depleted

- Modest bunch new coriander, chopped, in addition to extra for sprinkling
- 140g thick, unsweetened coconut yogurt

Technique:
1. Heat the oil in an enormous non-stick skillet and fry the onions for 8 mins until relaxed and brilliant. Add the ginger, garlic, bean stew and thyme and cook, blending, for 1 min. add the flavors, mix momentarily ridiculous, at that point pour in the tomatoes and bouillon, and mix in the peppers, yam and plantains. Cover and leave to stew for 30 mins.
2. Then, heat up the rice as indicated by pack guidelines. Mix the beans into the stew with the coriander and cook delicately for 10 mins until the peppers are delicate.
3. Spoon a large portion of the rice and stew into two dishes, top each with 2 tbsp. yogurt and dissipate with coriander, to serve. Cool the excess stew and rice, at that point cover and chill to eat on one more night with the leftover yogurt. To serve once more, delicately reheat the stew in a dish with a sprinkle of water until foaming. The rice can be reheated in the microwave.

4. Whole roasted cauliflower with anchovy sauce

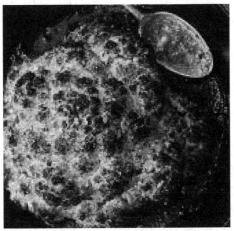

Prep: 20 mins Cook: 1 hr. Serves 4 – 6

Ingredients:

- 1whole huge cauliflower
- Olive oil, for showering
- 2 banana shallots, finely chopped
- 3 garlic cloves finely cut
- Great squeeze dried stew drops
- 8 salted anchovies, finely chopped
- 600g tomatoes, finely chopped
- 75ml vegetable stock
- 100ml twofold cream
- 50g salted spread

Strategy:

1. Heat oven to 200C/180C/gas 6. Eliminate the leaves from the cauliflower and put away to utilize later. Bring an enormous dish of salted

water to the bubble and whiten the cauliflower for 4-5 mins. Channel well.

2. Put the cauliflower in a simmering tin and sprinkle done with olive oil. Season well and dish for 40-50 mins until delicate and brilliant.

3. In the mean time, make the sauce. Shower a little oil in a dish and delicately fry the shallots for 10 mins until mollified. Add a large portion of the garlic and the stew chips and cook briefly more. Add the anchovies and let them break up; at that point add the tomatoes and stock.

4. Season and cook for 10-15 mins until the tomatoes have separated. Add the cream and air pocket for one more moment.

5. Heat the margarine in a different container with the remainder of the garlic and fry the cauliflower leaves with a lot of preparing. Serve the cauliflower on the rich leaves, with the anchovy sauce spooned over the top.

Works out in a good way for

Spanish omelet

Spanish sardines on toast

Spanish sticks

5. Gin & tonic cheesecake

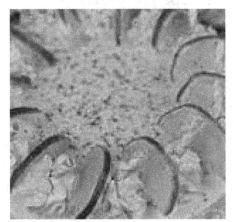

Prep: 25 mins Cook: 5 mins plus cooling and chilling overnight Serves 10-12

Ingredients:
- 250g stomach related bread rolls
- 100g margarine, softened
- 600g cream cheddar
- 100g icing sugar
- Zing and juice of 1 lime, in addition to additional zing to serve
- 50ml gin
- 280ml twofold cream
- 250ml can gin and tonic
- 2 tbsp. caster sugar
- 1 lemon, half squeezed, half finely cut
- 2 medium meringues, squashed

Technique:
1. Margarine and line a 23cm free lined tin with preparing material. Put the stomach related bread rolls in a plastic food sack and smash to

pieces using a moving pin, or barrage in a food processor. Move to a bowl; at that point pour over the dissolved margarine. Blend altogether until the scraps are totally covered. Tip them into the readied tin and press immovably down into the base to make an even layer. Chill in the ice chest for 1 hr. to set immovably.

2. To make the filling, place the cream cheddar, icing sugar and lime zing in a bowl, at that point beat with an electric rush until smooth. Tip in the gin and twofold cream, and keep beating until the blend is thick and totally consolidated. Presently spoon it onto the bread roll base, and spread to the edges. Smooth the highest point of the cheesecake down with the rear of a treat spoon or spatula. Leave to set in the refrigerator short-term.

3. Pour the container of gin and tonic into a dish, add the caster sugar and lemon squeeze and bubble hard. Whenever it has decreased to syrup (around 3-4 minutes over high heat), cool a little, at that point add the lime juice and the cuts of lemon and throw in the syrup. Permit to cool totally.

4. To serve, place the base of the cheesecake on top of a can; at that point slowly pull the sides of the tin down. Slip the cake onto a serving plate, eliminating the coating paper and base. Top with a small bunch of the squashed meringues; at that point sprinkle with the syrup, dispersing the lemon cuts on top as you go. Add a last cleaning of lime zing, cut and serve.

6. Dauphinoise potatoes

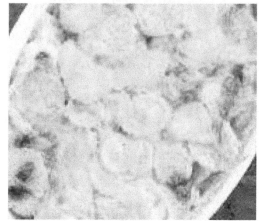

Prep: 30 mins Cook: 1 hr. and 10 mins Serves 8 – 10

Ingredients:
- 4 narrows leaves
- Bundle thyme
- 500ml twofold cream
- 500ml crème fraise
- A grinding of nutmeg
- 1 garlic clove, divided
- 50g margarine, in addition to extra for the dish
- 2 ½kg Maris Piper potatoes or Desiree potatoes, all generally a similar size, stripped

Technique:
1. Slam the cove and thyme, at that point put into a pan with the cream, crème fraîche, nutmeg and one portion of the garlic clove. Season liberally. Bring to the bubble; at that

point stew for 2 mins. Put away to cool and mix.

2. Heat oven to 180C/160C fan/gas 6. Sprinkle the cut side of the leftover portion of garlic with salt and use it to rub within a large rectangular gratin dish. Gently margarine the dish. Liquefy the excess margarine in a pot.

3. Daintily cut the potatoes using a mandoline and stack them in heaps. Firmly pack the stacks width ways in the dish, remaining on their side, using just as numerous as will cozily fill the dish. Strain the warm cream over the potatoes, pushing down on the spices as you do as such. Heat for 1 hr. or until the potatoes is cooked through and fresh on the top, brushing with the softened margarine part of the way through. Leave to cool for around 10 mins, at that point serve scooped directly from the dish.

Works out positively for

Broil chicken

Christmas turkey with clementine and straight margarine

Simple turkey crown

7. Bouillabaisse

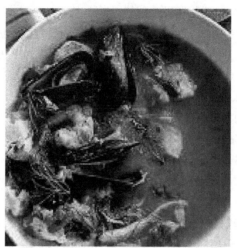

Prep: 1 hr. Cook: 1 hr. A challenge Serves 6
Ingredients:

- 1 leek, green upper left entire, white finely cut
- Little bundle new thyme
- 3 narrows leaves
- Bundle parsley, follows entire, leaves generally chopped
- 2 pieces of orange strip
- 1 gentle red bean stew
- 4 tbsp. olive oil
- 2 onions, chopped
- 1 leek
- 1 fennel, fronds picked and held, fennel chopped
- 4 garlic cloves, minced
- 1 tbsp. tomato purée
- 1 star anise
- 2 tbsp. Period, discretionary, on the off chance that you have it
- 4 large, ready tomatoes, chopped

- Large squeeze (⅓ tsp.) saffron strands
- 1 ½l fish stock
- 100g potato, one stripped piece
- 1kg of fileted blended Mediterranean fish, each filet cut into large lumps. (We utilized a blend of red and dark mullet, monkfish, John Dory and gurnard)
- 300g mussels, discretionary
- For the rouille
- 2 garlic cloves
- 1 little piece of red bean stew (discretionary)
- Little squeeze saffron
- 1 piece of potato, cooked in the stock, (see above)
- 1 egg yolk
- 100ml olive oil
- 1 tbsp. lemon juice
- For the bread garnishes
- ½ roll, daintily cut
- 1 tbsp. olive oil

Technique:

1. To make the bread garnishes heat oven to 200C/180C fan/gas 6. Lay the cuts of bread on a level preparing plate in a solitary layer shower with olive oil and heat for 15 mins until brilliant and fresh. Put away – can be made a day ahead and kept in a water/air proof holder.
2. Utilize a layer of the green piece of the leek to fold over and make a spice pack with the thyme, straight, parsley stalks, orange strip and stew. Tie everything along with kitchen string and put away.

3. Heat the oil in an exceptionally large meal dish or stock pot and toss in the onion, cut leek and fennel and cook for around 10 mins until mollified. Mix through the garlic and cook for 2 mins more, at that point add the spice group, tomato purée, star anise, Pernod if using, chopped tomatoes and saffron. Stew and mix briefly then pour over the fish stock. Season with salt and pepper, bring to a stew, and at that point add the piece of potato. Air pockets everything delicately for 30 mins until you have a flimsy tomatoes soup. At the point when that piece of potato is near the precarious edge of breakdown, fish it out and put away to make the rouille.

4. While the stock is stewing make the rouille by pounding the garlic, bean stew and saffron with a spot of salt in a mortar with a pestle. Squash in the cooked potato to make a tacky paste at that point speed in the egg yolk and, slowly, the olive oil until you make a mayonnaise-like sauce. Mix in the lemon squeeze and put away.

5. When the stout tomato stock has cooked you have two alternatives: for a provincial bouillabaisse, essentially poach your fish in it alongside the mussels, in case you're using (just until they open) and serve. For a refined rendition, eliminate the spice group and star anise. Using a handheld or table-top blender, barrage the soup until smooth. Pass the soup through a strainer into a large, clean dish and bring to a delicate stew. Beginning with the densest fish, add the lumps to the stock and

cook for 1 min prior to adding the following sort. With the fish we utilized, the request was: monkfish, John Dory, dim mullet, snapper. At the point when all the fish is in, dissipate over the mussels, if using, and stew everything for around 5 mins until just cooked and the mussels have opened.

6. Utilize an opened spoon to painstakingly scoop the fish and mussels out onto a warmed serving platter, soak with a tiny bit of stock and disperse over the chopped parsley. Carry everything to the table. A few group eat it as two courses, serving the stock with bread garnishes and rouille first, at that point the fish spooned into a similar bowl. Others basically serve it as a fish stew. However you pick the rouille is there to be mixed into the stock to thicken and give it a kick.

8. Alkaline Chili & orange salmon with watercress new potatoes & wasabi mayo

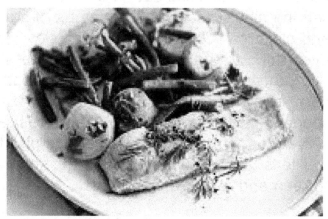

Prep: 20 mins Cook: 20 mins Serves 4-6
Ingredients:

- 2 oranges, both zested, 1 squeezed and 1 cut into cuts
- 1-2 red chilies, finely chopped
- 2 tbsp. sesame oil
- 2 garlic cloves, squashed
- 1 large or 2 more modest fennel bulbs finely cut (500g)
- 850g side of salmon, skin on
- 750g infant new potato, split assuming large
- 200g watercress, generally chopped
- 1 tbsp. additional virgin olive oil
- 100g mayonnaise
- 3-4 tsp. wasabi paste

Strategy:

1. Heat the oven to 200C/180C fan/gas 6. Whisk the vast majority of the orange zing and all the juice, stew, sesame oil and garlic in a little bowl, at that point season. Line a heating plate with foil, dissipate over the fennel and wrap up the greater part of the orange cuts. Add the salmon on top, skin-side down, pour over the sauce, and top with the remainder of the orange cuts. Cook in the oven for 20 mins or until flaky and cooked through.

2. Then, heat up the potatoes for 15 mins or until delicate. Channel and tip once again into the container. Add the majority of the watercress and the olive oil throws everything along with some flavoring and leave for a couple of mins for the watercress to wither.

3. Whisk together the mayo, wasabi and staying orange zing. Present with the salmon and potatoes, and dissipate over the excess watercress to serve.

Formula TIPS

SALMON Filets WORK TOO...

Utilize 4-6 salmon filets on the off chance that you can't get hold of a side of salmon. Push them together, so they take a similar measure of time in the oven, and look more noteworthy when taken to the table.

9. Melting middle onions

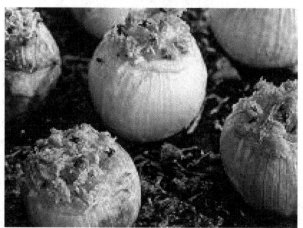

Prep: 50 mins Cook: 1 hr. and 45 mins Serves 4

Ingredients:

- 8 large brown onions
- 40g spread
- 70g pine nuts
- 150g delicate white breadcrumbs
- 1 garlic clove, finely ground
- 5 thyme twigs, leaves picked
- ½ little bundle of parsley, finely chopped
- 1 medium egg, beaten
- 100g scarmoza (smoked mozzarella) or customary mozzarella

Strategy:

1. Heat the oven to 180C/160C fan/gas 4. Cut a little plate off the root lower part of every onion so they stand upstanding. Cut 1cm cuts off the tops (these will be utilized as tops), at that point set back on top of the onions.

Enclose every onion by foil, move to a heating plate, and prepare for 1 hr. until delicate.

2. Liquefy the margarine in a container. Tip into a bowl. Add the pine nuts to the dish and toast over a low heat for 2 mins until brilliant. Add to the spread with the breadcrumbs, garlic, thyme, parsley and egg. Mix, at that point season.

3. Cut the cheddar into 8 stout blocks. At the point when the onions are adequately cool to deal with, scoop out the delicate focuses, leaving a couple of layers of onion at the edge. Finely slash the scooped-out focuses from 2 onions, and add to the breadcrumb blend (save the rest to use in another formula, for example, ragu). Spoon the breadcrumb combination into the emptied out onions so they're mostly full, at that point drive a piece of cheddar into the center of each and top up with more breadcrumb blend. Top every onion with its 'cover', at that point cook for 35-40 mins more until delicate and the cheddar is liquefied.

Works out in a good way for

Entire truffle cooks celeriac with cheddar sauce and hazelnuts

Simple veggie lover nut broil

Nectar broil beetroot and Wensleydale tart tartine

10. Squidgy chocolate pear pudding

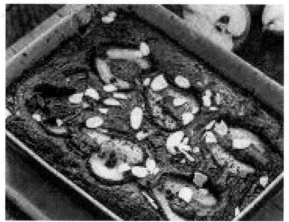

Prep: 20 mins Cook: 35 mins Serves 8

Ingredients:
- 200g spread, in addition to extra for lubing
- 300g brilliant caster sugar
- 4 large eggs
- 75g plain flour
- 50g cocoa powder
- 410g can pear parts in juice, depleted
- 100g plain dull chocolate (70% cocoa solids)
- 25g chipped almonds (discretionary)
- Cream or frozen yogurt, to serve

Strategy:
1. Heat oven to 190C/170C fan/gas 5. Daintily oil an approximately 20 x 30cm shallow ovenproof dish. Put the spread in a large pan and spot over a low heat until just softened. Eliminate the spread from the heat and mix in the sugar until all around consolidated.

2. Whisk the eggs together in a large bowl. Slowly add the eggs to the margarine and sugar, beating great with a wooden spoon in the middle of every option. Filter the flour and cocoa powder on top of the egg combination, at that point beat hard with a wooden spoon until altogether consolidated.
3. Fill the readied tin or dish and settle the pears into the chocolate player. Put the chocolate on a board and cut into thick pieces generally 1.5cm with a large blade. Disperse the chocolate pieces over the player and sprinkle with almonds, in the event that you like. Can be frozen at this stage.
4. Prepare in the focal point of the oven for 30 mins or until the blend is dried up on a superficial level and gently cooked inside. Try not to permit to overcook, as the cake will become elastic instead of gooey in the middle. Serve warm with cream or frozen yogurt

Formula TIPS

TO FREEZE

Wrap the cooled, unbaked pudding firmly in foil, name and freeze for as long as multi month. To serve, open up the pudding and heat from frozen as above in sync 4 for 50 mins.

Works out positively for

Extreme vanilla frozen yogurt

Cognac margarine frozen yogurt

11. Smashed chicken with corn slaw

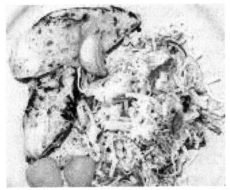

Prep: 10 mins Cook: 5 mins Serves 4

Ingredients:

- For the chicken
- 4 skinless chicken bosom filets
- 1 lime, zested and squeezed
- 2 tbsp. bio yogurt
- 1 tsp. new thyme leaves
- ¼ tsp. turmeric
- 2 tbsp. finely chopped coriander
- 1 garlic clove, finely ground
- 1 tsp. rapeseed oil
- For the slaw
- 1 little avocado
- 1 lime, zested and squeezed
- 2 tbsp. bio yogurt
- 2 tbsp. finely chopped coriander
- 160g corn, cut from 2 cobs
- 1 red pepper, deseeded and chopped
- 1 red onion, split and finely cut
- 320g white cabbage finely cut
- 150g new potatoes, bubbled, to serve

Strategy:
1. Slice the chicken breasts down the middle; at that point put them between two sheets of preparing material and slam with a moving pin to straighten. Blend the lime zing and juice with the yogurt, thyme, turmeric, coriander and garlic in a large bowl. Add the chicken and mix until very much covered. Leave to marinate while you make the slaw.
2. Crush the avocado with the lime squeeze and zing, 2 tbsp. yogurt and the coriander. Mix in the corn, red pepper, onion and cabbage.
3. Heat a large non-stick skillet or frying pan container, at t at point cook the chicken in clusters for a couple of mins each side – they'll cook rapidly as they're slender. Serve the hot chicken with the slaw and the new potatoes. In case you're cooking for two, chill a large portion of the chicken and slaw for lunch one more day (eat inside two days).

12. Miso noodles with fried eggs

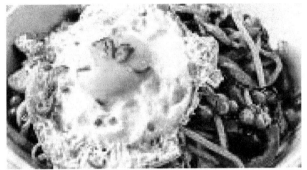

Prep: 10 mins Cook: 12 mins Serves 2

Ingredients

- 2 homes whole meal noodles (100g)
- 1 tbsp. rapeseed oil, in addition to a drop extra for fricasseeing
- 30g ginger, cut into matchsticks
- 1 green pepper, deseeded and cut into strips
- 2 leeks (165g) meagerly cut
- 3 large garlic cloves, finely ground
- 1 tsp. smoked paprika
- 1 tbsp. brown miso
- 160g beansprouts
- 100g frozen peas, thawed out
- 160g infant spinach
- 2 large eggs
- 1 red bean stew, deseeded and chopped (discretionary)

Technique:

1. Put the noodles in a bowl and cover with bubbling water. Put away to relax.

2. Then, heat the oil in a wok and sautéed food the ginger, pepper and leek for a couple of mins until relaxed. Add the garlic and paprika and cook for 1 min more. Channel the noodles, hold 2 tbsp. of the water and blend in with the miso.

3. Add the depleted noodles, miso fluid, beansprouts, peas and spinach to the wok and throw over a high heat until the spinach shrivels. While you are doing this, fry the eggs in a little oil however you would prefer. Heap the noodles onto plates, top with the eggs and bean stew, if using, and serve.

13. Vegan moussaka

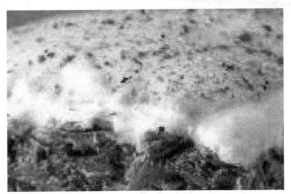

Prep: 40 mins Cook: 1 hr. and 45 mins Serves 6
Ingredients:

- 30g sack dried porcini mushrooms
- 8 tbsp. olive oil
- 1 onion, finely chopped
- 2 carrots, finely chopped
- 2 celery sticks, finely chopped
- 4 garlic cloves cut
- Hardly any springs of thyme
- 1 tsp. tomato purée
- 100ml vegetarian red wine (discretionary)
- 250g dried green lentils
- 2 x 400g jars entire plum tomatoes
- 250g pack chestnut mushrooms, chopped
- 250g pack Portobello mushrooms, cut
- 1 tsp. soy sauce
- 1 tsp. Marmite
- 1kg floury potato (like Maris Piper), stripped and chopped
- 1 ½ tsp. dried oregano
- 3 aubergines cut lengthways
- 150ml soya milk

Strategy:

1. Pour 800ml bubbling water over the dried porcini and leave for 10 mins until hydrated. In the interim, empty 1½ tbsp. oil into a large pan. Add the onion, carrot, celery and a spot of salt. Cook tenderly, mixing for 10 mins until delicate. Eliminate the porcini from the fluid, keeping the mushroomy stock and generally hack. Put both away.

2. Add the garlic and thyme to the skillet. Cook for 1 min, at that point mix in the tomato purée and cook briefly more. Pour in the red wine, on the off chance that using, cook until almost diminished, adds the lentils, held mushroom stock and tomatoes. Bring to the bubble; at that point diminish the heat and leave to stew with the cover on.

3. Then, heat a large griddle. Add 1½ tbsp. oil and tip the entirety of the mushrooms into the container, including the rehydrated ones. Fry until all the water has vanished and the mushrooms are profound brilliant brown. Pour in the soy sauce. Give everything a decent blend; at that point scratch the mushrooms into the lentil pot.

4. Mix in the Marmite, at that point keep on cooking the ragu, blending at times, over a low-medium heat for 30-45 mins until the lentils are cooked and the sauce is thick and diminished, adding additional water if essential. Eliminate the thyme twigs and season to taste.

5. Heat oven to 180C/160C fan/gas 4. Put the potatoes into a dish of cold salted water. Bring

to the bubble, at that point cook until mashable.

6. In the mean time, blend the leftover 5 tbsp. oil with the oregano, at that point brush the aubergine cuts with its majority and sprinkle with ocean salt. Iron for 3 mins on each side until delicate.

7. Channel and squash the potatoes with the soya milk. Season to taste.

8. Spoon the ragu into a large lasagna dish (or two more modest ovenproof dishes); layer in ½ the aubergine, trailed by the squash. Brush the excess oregano oil across the crush, at that point wrap up by fixing with the leftover aubergine cuts. Prepare in the oven for 25-35 mins until brilliant and percolating.

Works out positively for

Vegetarian ragu

Salted tomato salad

Bulgur wheat tabbouleh

14. Cheesy sausage & bean pies

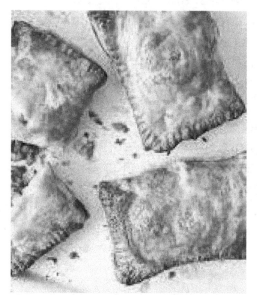

Prep: 25 mins Cook: 40 mins Serves 4

Ingredients:

- 400g can chop haricot beans, depleted and flushed
- 4 frankfurters, cooked, at that point cut into adjusts
- 150g passata
- Spot of dried oregano
- 4 spring onions, chopped
- Spot of sugar
- 320g prepared moved puff cake sheet
- 50g cheddar, ground
- 1 egg, beaten
- Salad, to serve

Technique:

1. Heat the oven to 200C/180C fan/gas 6. Join the beans, hotdogs, passata, oregano and spring onions with some flavoring and the sugar.
2. Unroll the cake and cut into four square shapes. Spoon the bean and frankfurter combination onto one side of every square shape, leaving a 1cm boundary – so you can overlay the cake like a book. Sprinkle the cheddar over the bean and hotdog combination.
3. Brush some egg around the edges; at that point overlay the cake over to encase the filling. Seal the edges by squeezing with a fork, at that point put on a preparing sheet fixed with heating material. Brush with more egg, and cut a little opening in the highest point of every pie for steam to get away. Will keep chilled for up to 24 hrs. Heat the oven to 180C/160C fan/gas 4.
4. Prepare on the center rack for 40 mins until brilliant. Leave to cool for 5 mins, at that point present with salad.

15. Sausage & pesto pizza

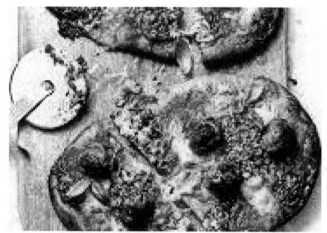

***Prep: 20 mins Cook: 40 mins plus defrosting
Serves 4***

Ingredients:

- 2 x 220g frozen pizza mixture
- 400g can chop tomatoes
- 3 pork wieners
- Glug of olive oil
- 6 tbsp. new pesto or vegan elective
- 2 x 125g balls wild ox mozzarella
- Basil leaves, to serve (discretionary)

Technique:

1. Eliminate the pizza mixture from the cooler 1-2 hrs. Prior to cooking to thaw out. Heat the oven to 220C/200C fan/gas 7. Put a large preparing sheet in the oven to heat.
2. Tip the chopped tomatoes into a pot, stew revealed for 15 mins until decreased and sassy, at that point season to taste.

3. Extract the sausage meat from the skins and into a bowl. Gap into 10 little balls. Empty the oil into a non-stick griddle and fry the meatballs over a medium heat for 5 mins until brilliant brown.
4. Carry the batter out into two oval-formed pizzas about 20cm long. Top with a layer of the pureed tomatoes; at that point twirl in the pesto. Tear the mozzarella and dissipate that over alongside the wiener meatballs. Slide the pizzas onto the hot preparing sheet and cook for 18-20 mins or until fresh and singed at the edges. Disperse over a couple of basil leaves to serve, in the event that you like.

Formula TIPS

MAKE THEM VEGGIE

Trade the frankfurters for relieved meats, on the off chance that you like, or Portobello mushroom cuts, on the off chance that you need them to be sans meat.

Works out in a good way for

Extreme pizza Marguerite

New potato and rosemary pizza

Pepper and fish Panini pizzas

16. Alkaline Breton braised lamb & haricot beans

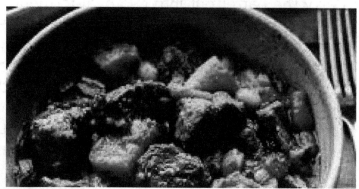

Prep: 20 mins Cook: 2 hrs. And 45 mins plus overnight soaking Serves 6
Ingredients:

- 250g haricot beans, doused for the time being and depleted
- 2 large onions, 1 generally chopped, 1 quartered
- 3 entire carrots, stripped, 1 divided lengthways, 2 diced
- 2 sticks celery, 1 divided, 1 diced
- 2 narrows leaves
- Bundle of parsley, stalks and leaves isolated, leaves chopped
- 6 dark peppercorns
- 2 tbsp. olive oil
- 1kg braising sheep (shoulder is acceptable), cut into pieces
- 4 garlic cloves, finely chopped
- 400g can cherry tomatoes
- 1 tbsp. tomato purée

- 400ml sheep stock or chicken stock

Strategy:
1. Put the beans in a pot and cover with water. Add the quartered onion, the split carrot and divided celery, the sound leaves, parsley stalks and peppercorns. Bring to the bubble, diminish the heat and stew for 30-40 mins until the beans are delicate. Channel well and hold the cooking fluid, disposing of the onion, carrot and celery.
2. While the beans are cooking, heat a large portion of the olive oil in a substantial based flameproof meal. Brown the sheep in groups over a high heat. As each cluster is cooked, eliminate it and put away on a plate. Decrease the heat, add the chopped onion to the container with the diced celery and carrot and cook until very much shaded. Add the garlic and cook for several mins.
3. Return the sheep to the skillet and add every one of the leftover ingredients, with the exception of the beans. Bring to the bubble, diminish the heat to exceptionally low and cover, at that point cook for 2 hrs. Add the beans 45 mins before the finish of cooking time. Mix the sheep round from time to time. On the off chance that the sheep looks dry, add a portion of the bean cooking fluid.
4. Eliminate the top for the last 30 mins of cooking time, and season. This aides the cooking fluid to lessen. You should wind up with a thick stew of delicate sheep and delicate beans. Dissipate over the parsley and serve.

Works out positively for

Wild garlic margarine

Carrot and yam pound

17. Smoky hake, beans & greens

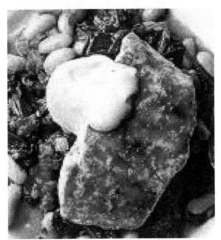

Prep: 15 mins Cook: 10 mins Serves 2

Ingredients:

- Gentle olive oil
- ½ x 200g pack crude cooking chorizo (we utilized Unearthed Alfresco Smoked)
- 1 onion, finely chopped
- 260g sack spinach
- 2 x 140g skinless hake filets
- ½ tsp. sweet smoked paprika
- 1 red bean stew, deseeded and shredded
- 400g can cannellini beans, depleted
- Juice ½ lemons
- 1 tbsp. additional virgin olive oil
- To serve
- Speedy garlic mayonnaise (optional) - see formula in tip

Strategy:

1. Heat up a full pot of water and heat the flame broil to high. Heat 1 tsp. oil in a large skillet. Press the meat from the chorizo straightforwardly into the container. Add the onion and fry for 5 mins, smashing the meat with a spatula until separated, brilliant and encompassed by its juices. The onion will likewise be delicate and brilliant.
2. In the interim, put the spinach in a colander, gradually pour over the bubbled water to shrivel it, and at that point run under the virus tap. Press out the abundance water using your hands, at that point put away. Line a preparing plate with foil, rub with a little oil and spot the fish on top. Season, sprinkle over the smoked paprika and shower with somewhat more oil.
3. Tip the stew into the container with the hotdogs, fry for 1 min more, and at that point add the beans, spinach, lemon juice and additional virgin olive oil. Allow it to warm through tenderly, at that point season to taste.
4. Barbecue the fish for 5 mins or until flaky however not dry – you will not have to turn it. Spoon the bean combination onto plates, at that point cautiously top with the fish and any juices from the plate. Present with a spot of Quick garlic mayonnaise (see formula, right), on the off chance that you like.

Formula TIPS

Fast GARLIC MAYONNAISE

Add 2 egg yolks to a medium bowl with the zing 1 lemon, 2 tsp. every lemon juice and Dijon mustard, 1 little squashed garlic clove and some flavoring. Beat with electric hand blenders until consolidated – at that point, beating persistently, gradually stream in 200ml gentle olive oil to make a thick, plush mayonnaise. On the off chance that you add it excessively fast, the sauce will part, so fare thee well. Season and add somewhat more lemon juice if necessary. In the event that it tastes right however feels all in all too thick, release with a little water. Cover and chill. Will keep for as long as 3 days.

Works out in a good way for

Mustardy greens

Stoved potatoes

Green beans with shallots

18. Tear-and-share cheese & garlic rolls

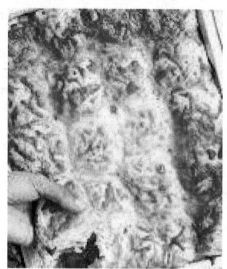

Prep: 40 mins Cook: 40 mins Plus as least 2 hrs. Proving Makes 20

Ingredients:

- 100g unsalted margarine , relaxed
- 450g solid white bread flour
- 7g sachet quick activity dried yeast
- 1 tsp. brilliant caster sugar
- rapeseed oil , for the bowl and plate
- 2 tbsp. polenta or cornmeal
- 1 garlic clove , ground
- 100g mozzarella , ground
- 50g cheddar , ground

Technique:

1. Heat 280ml water in a pan briefly until warm however not very hot to put your finger in (don't consume yourself!). Eliminate from the

heat, at that point add 50g spread. Join the flour, yeast, sugar and 1 tsp. salt in a large bowl or a tabletop blender. Add the warm water and beat to make a delicate batter. Work for 10 mins by hand, or 5 mins in a blender, until the batter feels stretchy and smooth. Tip into a perfect, oiled bowl and cover with oiled stick film. Leave to ascend for 1½-2 hrs. or until multiplied in size.

2. Brush a large preparing plate with oil and disperse over the polenta. Take the air out of the batter. Squeeze off little pieces (about the size of a pecan), at that point fold each piece into a ball and put on the preparing plate. Leave a little space between every batter ball.

3. Heat oven to 180C/160C fan/gas 4. Cover the plate with oiled stick film, at that point demonstrate for 30 mins-1 hr. until the mixture has multiplied in size and the balls are contacting. Blend the leftover spread in with the garlic. At the point when the rolls are prepared to cook, brush the tops with the garlic spread and disperse with the cheeses. Prepare for 25-30 mins until the batter balls are cooked through. Leave to cool for 5 mins, at that point serve.

Works out positively for

Lemon and yogurt chicken flatbreads

Bar-b-que chorizo potato salad

Pineapple and pork sticks

19. Noodle stir-fry with crunchy peanuts

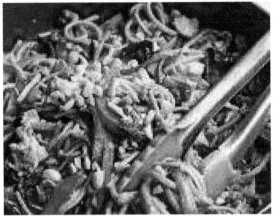

Prep: 10 mins Cook: 10 mins Serves 3

Ingredients:

- 2 tbsp. crunchy peanut butter
- 1 tbsp. soy sauce
- 1 tbsp. broiled unsalted peanuts , chopped, in addition to extra to serve
- 300g pack prepared to eat egg noodles
- 1 tbsp. oil
- 2 eggs , softly beaten
- 300g pack pan sear vegetables
- sweet stew sauce , to serve (optional)

Strategy:

1. Blend the peanut butter in with the soy sauce and 50ml water; at that point add the peanuts. Put the noodles in a bowl and cover them with bubbling water. Mix them tenderly so they independent, at that point channel.
2. Heat ½ tbsp. oil in a wok or large griddle, and pour in the egg. Leave the egg to set, at that

point hack it up with your spatula and tip it onto a plate. Heat the excess oil in the wok. Sautéed food the veg until beginning to shrivel, at that point add the noodles and continue to cook. Return the egg to the wok, at that point spoon in the nut blend and throw. Split between bowls; at that point sprinkle over more peanuts. Present with sweet stew sauce, in the event that you like.

Works out positively for

Chicken and chickpea rice

Corn and prawn chowder

Pick and blend omelet in with crunchy bread garnishes

20. Kale & quinoa patties

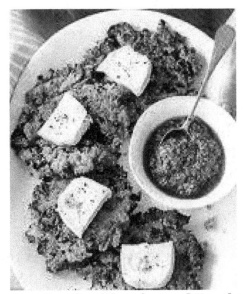

Prep: 30 mins Cook: 30 mins - 35 mins Serves 4

Ingredients:

- 140g quinoa
- 500g hot vegetable stock
- 100g kale , stalks eliminated, leaves generally chopped
- 3 tbsp. olive oil
- 1 little onion , finely chopped
- 2 garlic cloves , squashed
- 75g new white breadcrumbs
- 2 medium eggs , beaten
- 50g sundried tomatoes , generally chopped
- 100g goat's cheddar , cut from a round log
- green plate of mixed greens , to serve (optional)
- For the pesto
- ½ little pack basil , leaves as it were

- ½ little pack parsley , leaves as it were
- 2 garlic cloves , squashed
- 50g pine nuts , toasted
- 50g parmesan , ground
- 150g olive oil
- juice 1 lemon

Strategy:
1. Put the quinoa in a pot and pour over the hot stock. Stew for 18-20 mins over a delicate heat until the grains have lightened up and the fluid has vanished. Eliminate from the heat and permit to cool. Then, carry a large pan of water to the bubble. Add the kale and stew for 6-8 mins until cooked through. Channel, crush out any abundance water and put away.
2. Put 1 tbsp. olive oil in a little griddle over a medium heat. Add the onion and cook for 2-3 mins until clear. Add the garlic and cook for 1 min more. Tip the cooked quinoa into a bowl and add the kale, onion, garlic, breadcrumbs, egg and sundried tomatoes. Season well and blend to join. Put away.
3. To make the pesto, put the basil, parsley, garlic, pine nuts and Parmesan in a little food processor. Heartbeat, gradually pouring in the oil, until you have a thick pesto. Press in the lemon juice to release, at that point put away.
4. Tenderly heat 2 tbsp. olive oil in a shallow griddle. Using your hands, structure the quinoa combination into 8 round patties. Add to the skillet and fry for 4-5 mins each side until fresh and brilliant.

5. Heat the flame broil to high and put a cut of goat's cheddar on top of every patty. Spot under the flame broil to brown and dissolve the cheddar marginally – this will require only seconds, so watch out for them. Top every patty with a liberal spoonful of pesto and present for certain new green leaves, on the off chance that you like.

Works out in a good way for

Spiced yam wedges

Nursery salad

Quinoa salad with flame broiled halloumi

21. Turkey enchiladas

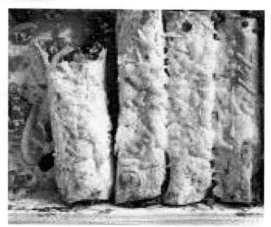

Prep: 20 mins Cook: 30 mins Serves 4
Ingredients:
- 1 tbsp. sunflower oil
- 500g turkey mince (2% fat)
- 1 medium onion, finely chopped
- 1 yellow pepper, deseeded and daintily cut
- 400g can chopped tomatoes
- 400g can red kidney beans in stew sauce
- 1 tbsp. new lime or lemon juice
- 2 stored tbsp. generally chopped coriander, in addition to extra to embellish
- 6 normal or 8 small scale flour tortillas
- 50g decreased fat develop cheddar, coarsely ground
- large blended plate of mixed greens, to serve

Strategy:
1. Heat oven to 200C/180C fan/gas 6. Heat the greater part of the oil in a large non-stick griddle. Fry the turkey, onion and pepper for 5 mins, blending consistently and separating the

mince with a wooden spoon. Add the chopped tomatoes and kidney beans.

2. Bring to a delicate stew and cook for 10 mins, blending consistently. Eliminate from the heat and mix in the lime juice and coriander. Season well.

3. Delicately oil a shallow ovenproof dish with the leftover oil. Put 1 tortilla in the dish and top two or three liberal spoonful's of the turkey combination. Move up and push aside of the dish. Rehash with different tortillas, at that point spoon any leftover turkey combination down the sides of the dish.

4. Sprinkle the tortillas with the cheddar and heat for 15 mins. Disperse coriander over the enchiladas and present with a serving of mixed greens.

Works out in a good way for

Avocado and bean stew salad

Pico de Gallo

Crunchy corn and pepper salsa

22. Lebanese-style meatballs with mujadara

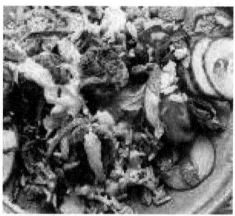

Prep: 15 mins Cook: 55 mins plus chilling
Serves 4
Ingredients:
- 250g sheep mince (10% fat or lower)
- 2 large onions (320g), 1 finely chopped, 1 divided and meagerly cut
- 1 garlic clove , finely ground
- 3 tsp. ground cumin
- 1 lemon , half zested and squeezed, half slice into four wedges to serve
- 2 tsp. rapeseed oil
- 200g brown basmati rice
- 1 tbsp. bouillon powder
- 390g can green lentils , depleted
- 2 tbsp. tahini
- For the plate of mixed greens
- 4 tomatoes , cut into wedges
- ¼ cucumber (about 150g), cut

- 12 Kalamata olives , quartered
- 1 tbsp. chopped mint , in addition to a couple of little leaves to serve

Strategy:
1. Tip the sheep into a bowl with ¼ of the chopped onion, the garlic, ½ tsp. cumin, the lemon zing and some dark pepper. Blend well in with your hands, at that point shape into 16 little meatballs. Chill for in any event 30 mins.
2. Heat 1 tsp. oil in a non-stick griddle over a medium-high heat. Hold the majority of the leftover chopped onion for the plate of mixed greens, at that point fries the rest for 5 mins until brilliant. Mix in the leftover cumin, at that point tip in the rice, bouillon powder, 500ml water and some dark pepper. Decrease the heat to a stew, at that point cover and cook over a medium heat for 30 mins. Tip in the lentils, cover again and cook for 5-10 mins more until the rice is delicate and all the water has been consumed.
3. In the interim, heat the leftover oil in a non-stick container over a medium-high heat. Add the meatballs and cut onion, cover and cook for 5 mins. Mix, at that point cook for 5 mins more until the meatballs are cooked through and the onions are brilliant. Mix the tahini and lemon squeeze along with 3-4 tbsp. water to make a sauce.
4. Blend the entirety of the plate of mixed greens ingredients in with the saved chopped onion. In case you're following our Healthy Diet Plan, partition half of the mujadara between two

plates and top with half of the meatballs and onions. Spoon over portion of the tahini sauce and present with half of the plate of mixed greens, two lemon wedges and a couple of mint leaves. Cover and chill the excess bits to eat one more day. Will save for a few days in the ice chest.

23. Caramelised apple parfait with cinnamon toffee sauce

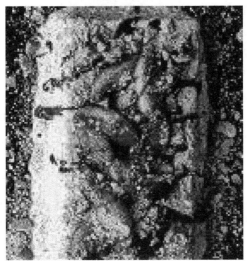

Prep: 40 mins Cook: 10 mins plus freezing a challenge Serves 8-10

Ingredients:
- For the parfait
- 6 Granny Smith apples , stripped, cored and cut into eighths
- 150g demerara sugar
- 100ml liquor
- 3 eggs
- 125g caster sugar
- 150ml twofold cream
- 10 digestive bread rolls , squashed, to serve
- For the cinnamon toffee sauce
- 200g dim brown delicate sugar
- 25g margarine , chopped
- 50ml twofold cream

- 50ml shady squeezed apple
- ½ tsp. ground cinnamon

Technique:
1. Tip the apples, demerara sugar and liquor into a container, bring to the bubble and stew for 12-15 mins until caramelized and tacky, at that point leave to cool. Scoop about 33% of the wedges out of the sauce and put away, at that point utilize a blender or food processor to purée the remainder of the apples and sauce, at that point put away.
2. Separate the eggs and tip the yolks into a large metal bowl. Put away the whites for some other time. Disintegrate 100g of the caster sugar in a medium pot with 120ml bubbling water. At the point when clear, bring to the bubble and put a sugar thermometer in the dish. Then, whisk the yolks in a bowl with an electric blender until velvety. At the point when the sugar syrup arrives at 120C, eliminate from the heat without a moment's delay. With the blender running, sprinkle the syrup onto the yolks and beat, on max throttle for 3-5 mins until you have a firm yellow froth. Leave to cool, whisking periodically.
3. Whisk the egg whites in a perfect bowl with a spotless rush until they structure firm pinnacles, at that point race in portion of the excess caster sugar and keep on racing for 30 seconds, at that point add the remainder of the sugar and keep racing until hardened pinnacles have framed once more. In a third bowl, whisk the cream until delicate pinnacles structure.

Tenderly crease the apple purée through the egg yolk combination, at that point overlay that through the egg whites and ultimately overlap that blend through the whipped cream. Continue collapsing until everything is completely consolidated. Fill a 900g portion tin fixed with stick film and freeze for the time being. Can be made fourteen days ahead of time and kept frozen.

4. To make the sauce, tip the sugar and margarine into a pan and heat until it begins to dissolve. When the sugar starts to bubble, add the cream, water, squeezed apple and cinnamon, cook out briefly, and at that point cool to room temperature. At the point when prepared to serve, turn out the parfait, top with the saved apple wedges and the digestive scraps; at that point sprinkle over the toffee sauce.

24. Campfire smoky bean brekkie

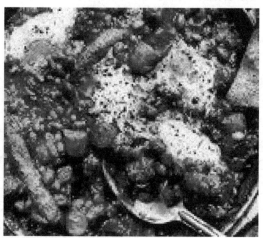

Prep: 10 mins Cook: 30 mins Serves 8-10 (easily halved)

Ingredients:

- 4 tbsp. olive or rapeseed oil
- 3-4 rosemary twigs
- 6 chipolatas
- 12 little cooking chorizo , divided
- 6 great quality smoked wiener hotdogs , cut into large pieces
- 2 onions , chopped
- 500ml container passata
- 300g great quality BBQ sauce (we utilized Stokes)
- 2 x 400g jars borlotti beans , depleted
- 2 x 400g jars haricot beans , depleted
- 8-10 eggs
- toast , to serve

Strategy:

1. Heat the oil in a large paella dish (our own was 45cm). Add the rosemary and sizzle briefly or 2 at that point scoop it out to a plate and put away. Add the chipolatas and brown all finished, push aside of the dish and add different wieners. Cook for a couple of mins until the chorizo begins to deliver a portion of its oil, at that point shoves these to the aside as well. Add the onions and cook until delicate, around 8 mins.
2. Add the passata, BBQ sauce and some flavoring, bring to a stew and air pocket for a couple of mins, at that point mix in the beans and take everything back to an air pocket.
3. Using the rear of a spoon, make little spaces in the beans and break in the eggs, spotting them over the surface. Cover the container with foil and cook delicately for 10 mins or until the eggs are cooked as you would prefer. Top with the rosemary and present with buttered toast and cups of tea.

Works out positively for

Pit fire cupcakes

One-dish English breakfast

On-the-run breakfast bars

25. Garlicky mushroom penne

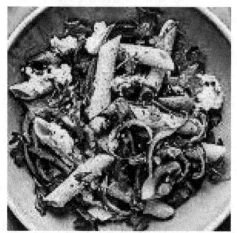

Prep: 20 mins Cook: 15 mins Serves 2
Ingredients:
- 210g can chickpeas , no compelling reason to deplete
- 1 tbsp. lemon juice
- 1 large garlic clove
- 1 tsp. vegetable bouillon
- 2 tsp. tahini
- ¼ tsp. ground coriander
- 115g whole meal penne
- 2 tsp. rapeseed oil
- 2 red onions , divided and cut
- 200g shut cup mushrooms , generally chopped
- ½ lemon , squeezed
- liberal modest bunch chopped parsley

Technique:
1. To make the hummus, tip a 210g can chickpeas with the fluid into a bowl and add 1

tbsp. lemon juice, 1 large garlic clove, 1 tsp. vegetable bouillon, 2 tsp. tahini and ¼ tsp. ground coriander.

2. Barrage to a wet paste with a hand blender, actually holding some surface from the chickpeas.

3. Cook 115g whole meal penne pasta as indicated by the pack guidelines.

4. Then, heat 2 tsp. rapeseed oil in a non-stick wok or large griddle and add 2 divided and cut red onions and 200g generally chopped shut cup mushrooms, blending often until mollified and beginning to caramelize.

5. Throw together softly, crush over the juice of ½ a lemon and serve, adding a scramble of water to relax the combination a little if necessary. Disperse with a liberal small bunch of chopped parsley.

26. Indian sweet potato & dhal pies

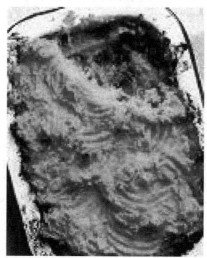

Prep: 15 mins Cook: 25 mins Serves 2

Ingredients:

- 650g yams , stripped and cut into little lumps
- 1 onion , split and daintily cut
- 2 carrots , scoured, divided and cut lengthways
- 15g ginger , finely ground
- 2 garlic cloves , finely ground
- 2 tsp. oil
- 1 tbsp. curry powder
- 1 vegetable stock 3D shape
- 2 tbsp. tomato purée
- 85g red lentils
- great small bunch coriander , chopped, in addition to branches to serve
- liberal spoonful 0% fat Greek-style yogurt
- broccoli , to serve (optional)

Technique:

1. Spot the yam in a container of bubbling water and cook for 15 mins, or until delicate.
2. Then, heat the oil in a container and fry the onion and carrot, for 2 minutes, at that point add the garlic and ginger and cook, blending for 1 min more. Tip in the curry powder, mix round the skillet at that point add 750ml of the bubbling water with the stock 3D square, tomato purée and lentils. Cover the dish and bubble for 20 mins until the vegetables are delicate and the fluid has been retained. Mix in the chopped coriander.
3. At the point when the yams are cooked, channel and crush them with the yogurt and preparing.
4. Spoon the lentil blend into one major or two individual dishes at that point top with the yam combination, disperse with the coriander and present with broccoli, in the event that you like.

Formula TIPS

TO FINISH

Pop the dish under a hot barbecue for a couple of moments directly toward the finish to bronze the potatoes and add some heat.

Works out positively for

Egg and rocket pizzas

Porridge with blueberry compote

27. Maple, apple & pecan cake

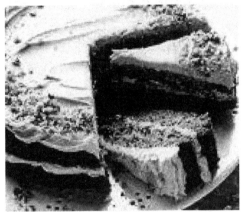

Prep: 30 mins Cook: 40 mins Serves 10

Ingredients:

- For the cake
- 115g spread , at room temperature
- 75g light brown delicate sugar
- 75ml maple syrup (the most obscure you can discover)
- 1 large egg , at room temperature, daintily beaten
- 225g plain flour , filtered
- 1½ tsp. bicarbonate of pop
- 1 tsp. preparing powder
- 100g walnuts , chopped
- 225g apple purée
- For the buttercream icing
- 125g spread
- 290g brilliant icing sugar
- 4 tbsp. dull maple syrup
- To brighten
- 30g walnuts

- 1 tbsp. delicate light brown sugar

Strategy:
1. To make the apple purée, cook 250g stripped and chopped cooking apples with a sprinkle of water in a container with a top until delicate for around 10 mins. Purée with a hand blender or in the little bowl of a food processor.
2. Spread and line the base of a 20cm spring form cake tin with material. Heat oven to 180C/160C fan/gas 4. Beat the spread and sugar until light and cushy. Blend the maple syrup and egg together and continuously add them. Filter the flour with the biker and preparing powder. Add a decent touch of salt and the nuts. With a large metal spoon, overlap the flour into the margarine and sugar, substituting with the apple purée. Scratch the player into the readied tin. Prepare for 40 mins, or until a stick embedded into the middle confesses all. Cool in the tin, at that point turn out onto a rack and strip off the heating material.
3. To make the buttercream, beat the spread until delicate, at that point add the icing sugar and beat until smooth. Step by step add the maple syrup, beating as you do as such. Cut the cooled cake fifty-fifty at that point, using a spatula, spread portion of the icing over the primary layer. Add the other layer on top, at that point top with the remainder of the buttercream. Heartbeat the walnuts in a food processor with the brown sugar (or finely hack

and blend). You should wind up with a coarse combination. Dissipate this over the highest point of the cake.

28. Hand-cut pappardelle

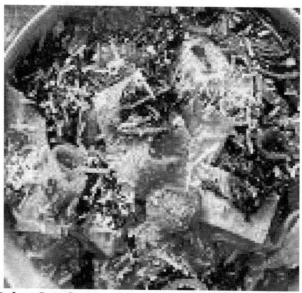

Prep: 1 hr.Cook:5 mins plus 1 hr. chilling
Serves 6-8
Ingredients:
- 750g '00' pasta flour
- 5 entire large eggs and 6 large egg yolks, both daintily beaten
- semolina flour , for cleaning
- You will require
- a pasta machine

Strategy:
1. Tip the '00' flour into a large food processor with a touch of salt and the beaten eggs and yolks. Heartbeat in short blasts, being mindful so as not to overheat the engine, and scratch the sides with a spatula between heartbeats to

fuse any dry flour. Quit beating when the blend has met up in even pieces. Tip onto a work surface and massage for 5-10 mins until you have a smooth, firm batter. In the event that it's actual dry, you may have to add a sprinkle of water to unite it. Shape into a ball, wrap and chill for in any event 1 hr. and as long as two days.

2. Keeping the remainder of the mixture very much covered; fold a quarter into a square shape that will fit through the most stretched out setting on your pasta machine. Pass the mixture through the machine, decreasing the width down to even out three. This implies it will not be really slight, yet will have a pleasant nibble to it when cooked.

3. Unfurl the mixture onto a work surface tidied with semolina. Cut it into more modest 25cm sheets, at that point cut every one of the sheets lengthways into 2.5cm-thick pappardelle strips. Throw the strips in semolina. Rehash the rolling and cutting with the excess batter, a quarter at a time. When all cut, leave to dry for a couple of mins on a material fixed plate liberally cleaned with semolina – this will make it simpler to deal with. Cook the pasta in a large dish of salted water for 3 mins, at that point channel to serve.

Conclusion

Lastly, I hope you liked all recipes in this book. Alkaline diet recipes add to more health benefits. Try these delicious recipes at home and appreciate along with your family.

CPSIA information can be obtained
at www.ICGtesting.com
Printed in the USA
LVHW011243060621
689455LV00002B/40